I0220754

Keeping Mobile
on
Your Scooter

By: Morris Barwick

Keeping Mobile on Your Scooter

ISBN: 10: 0615469051
ISBN-13: 978-0615469058 (Telar Sales Co)

DEDICATION

With all my love to my long suffering wife, Ann who has pushed, pulled, loaded and unloaded my scooters over the years.

Keeping Mobile on Your Scooter

CONTENTS

About the Author

ACKNOWLEDGMENTS

Many thanks to Johnny Stringer for the informational help, physical help, repair help and our Brainstorming sessions about Scooters.

PREFACE

In this book you will find my honest opinions without bias because I am not a distributor nor am I an affiliate of any mobility scooter or accessories industry.

After riding a scooter since 1988 for fun and now for necessity, I still find it fun. Hopefully, the things I present in this book will help to keep you "*On the trail and forked end down*" for many years to come.

Even though riding since 1988, I am still learning. Both beginner and experienced riders will recognize some of my experiences and profit from some of my mistakes and observations.

I am in the process of forming a club whereby we can share past and future experiences. Watch for:

http://www.mobilityscooterclub.com

CHAPTER 1
INTRODUCTION

It has been recently discovered that the 19 year old Egyptian King Tut had a bone disease and a foot and was severely affected. In his tomb were many sticks, obviously used in walking assistance. All of his wealth would never get what you have, convenient pain free personal mobility.

Allan R. Thieme invented the first mobility scooter in 1968 , being motivated to create this product to help a family member diagnosed with multiple sclerosis. It was a front wheel, chain drive that inspired the Amigo Corporation.

Today we have electrically powered wheelchairs and scooters making the occupant, or rider, totally independent of someone else's assistance. I know it can be a shock to find that your ability to walk has ended, is ending or will end. After 73 years, mine tapered off to non-walking but I find it is almost as great having wheels as walking. I am not claiming riding a scooter is better than walking, the only time that might be true is at fairs, flea markets and arenas. When standing in line, a scooter can be a big plus. My message to you is that:

You have not sacrificed your dignity.

It is rare that people stare, and when they do most of the time they are thinking "I wish I had one of those". Many times, I have heard the comment "That is what I need".

So welcome to the world of electrically powered personal transportation. Just relax, you will enjoy it! I present myself as an expert based on experience and engineering training. You will soon find things I have overlooked.

CHAPTER 2
GENERAL SCOOTER TYPES
AND SELECTION CONSIDERATIONS

A. **Large vs. small.** Unless you do a lot of distance riding, a large scooter can be an inconvenience. As a rule 4 MPH is an acceptable minimum. The smaller scooters seldom go above 5 MPH and are best used indoors.

B. **Will it go through my doors and maneuver around corners?** You should measure the opening going into all rooms you will be using, especially the bathroom. The width across the tires should be one inch, or more less than the door width. See discussion chapter for a hinge to add 2" width to any doorway.

C. **Does it separate into convenient parts for loading into the car?** If it will be rare that you take the scooter from home, it may be worth the occasional chore of disassembly, loading into the trunk and reassembly at your destination. Otherwise, see my chapter on transporting. There I will discuss the various means of lifting, or hoisting scooters for transporting with or in a vehicle.

D. **Four wheel vs. three wheel.** The main consideration here is that a three wheel can tip sideways easier, although with great difficulty, than a four wheeler. Tipping over can be caused by reaching too far to the side or travelling across an excessive slope without leaning uphill.

E. The three wheel scooter generally has a smaller turning radius that can be very important for an indoor scooter.

F.   **Solid tires or pneumatic tires.** You do not need to be somewhere with a flat tire. Pneumatic tires are intended for smoother riding, but I have never felt it worth the risk. I have not sensed a smoother ride from them. Get solid tires.

G.   **Springs in suspension.** To my knowledge of available scooters a spring suspension is only in the bigger scooters and rarely there. Leaf springs are in my Rascal. The Rascal rides so much smoother on our large rock driveway than either my: Pride, Amigo, Dalton, Sonic, Access Point Medical or Hoveround.

A COMMENT ON THE TRAILING WHEELS TYPE OF DESIGN.

The scooters that have the main wheels below the rider and have trailer wheels out back can present a new challenge to riding. In order to turn, the rear wheels go the opposite direction in order that you be headed in your desired direction. If you are near a wall on the right and decide to start up and go to the left, the scooter rotates to the left, causing the rear wheels to swing right and impact the wall. You have to allow for the extra length when making turns. My Hoveround was a fine scooter, able to be controlled by a joystick and **can drive the occupant up to a table as if sitting in a chair**. Hoveround has both three and four wheel designs available. My Hoveround had the trailing wheels design.

http://www.hoveround.com/

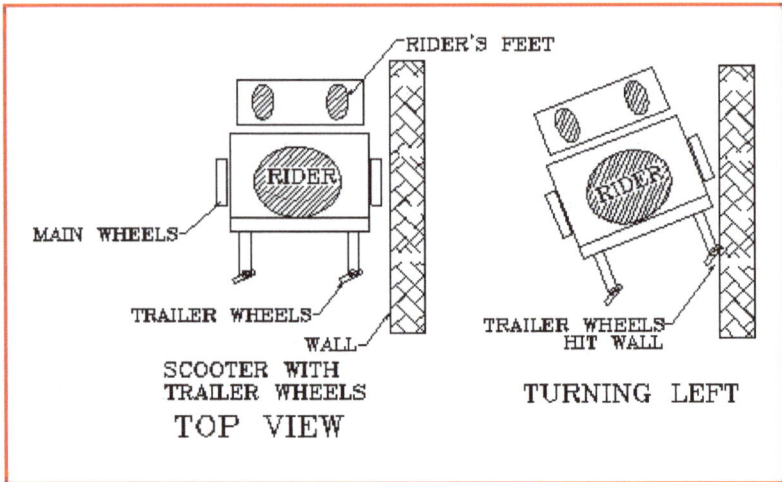

RIDER'S FEET

MAIN WHEELS

TRAILER WHEELS

WALL

SCOOTER WITH
TRAILER WHEELS
TOP VIEW

TRAILER WHEELS
HIT WALL

TURNING LEFT

A SCOOTER WITH REAR TRAILER WHEELS

Selection considerations assistance:

WHAT WILL THE SCOOTER BE USED FOR?

1. **Do you need longer range?** Then it will be a larger scooter, unless you purchase a spare battery pack to take with you
2. **Church?** I ride my three wheel PRIDE Sonic and sometimes my four wheel PRIDE Victory, pictured below. It is a pleasant ½ mile and I park in the aisle.

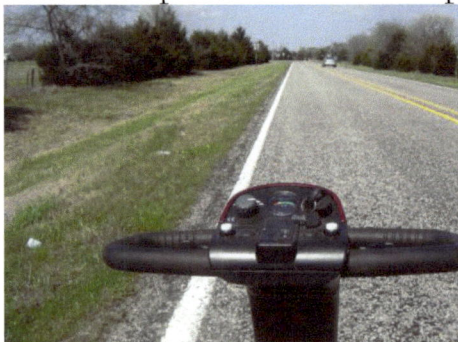

3. **In a house with limited space?**   Three wheel is best.
4. **In a house with generous space?**   Three wheel recommended but four wheel is O.K.
5. **In firm yard?** Three wheel or four wheel is O.K.
6. **In soft yard?** Four wheel is recommended
7. **Short neighborhood drives.** Three wheel or four wheel equally desirable.
8. **Flea markets or Carnivals?** Three wheels. Four wheels are harder to transport but usually have a longer range.
9. **Auditoriums and Arenas**, usually have a wheelchair section. Parking in the aisle is usually prohibited by fire regulations. A three wheel will eliminate any unsuspected maneuvering obstacles.

10. **Airline Travel?** I have travelled by air many times with my 138 pound Rascal, three wheel or my 85 pound Sonic three wheel. Usually you can ride down the jet way to the aircraft door. From there, you either walk to your seat or they take you in a narrow aisle wheelchair.
Then they take your scooter down the jet way stairway to be put into the baggage area. They are not responsible for damage, I have never had any serious damage.
When I get to my destination, sometime they take the scooter to baggage claim, whereupon they will wheelchair me to baggage claim. Other times, they will bring the scooter to the door of the plane for me. There is no charge to take the scooter.

CHAPTER 3
RIDER QUALIFICATIONS IN SCOOTER SELECTION

Is the rider able to steer using both the handle bars and throttle paddles with the needed manual dexterity to control speed and direction?

> If not, a joystick controlled scooter might be a better choice..

Can the rider sit erect, unaided?

> If so then the rider is a good candidate for a scooter

Does the rider have extremely limited sight?

> If so, then you should probably consider a manual wheelchair.

Can the rider walk at all, say into the bathroom from a large scooter outside in the hall?

> If so, width is not as great a consideration. This also makes four wheel less of an indoor hindrance. My preference is still three wheel.

Does the rider have a severe back condition that would be aggravated by a bumpy ride?

> If so, consult your doctor on advisability of riding a scooter instead of a powered wheel chair.. Even powered wheelchairs can give a bumpy ride. Take a look at the Electric Mobility Rascals with leaf spring suspension.

CHAPTER 4
SCOOTERS ON THE MARKET

(See more details in the Discussion section)

(Be sure to check out a "boogie Board" for use to transfer from bed to wheelchair, wheelchair to bath and wheelchair to automobile. The Beasy Transfer Boards use a frictionless bearing system for smooth, easy sliding with swivel a seat for greatest flexibility. I have used this and it was a blessing. 866-722-4581)

(Notice leaf spring suspension in the rear). Sharp turns at excessive speeds will also induce tipping. You will be offered the option of a power telescoping chair post. I have one on my Rascal. I find it only occasionally useful. One thing it does do is enable you to back up to the kitchen sink, rotate the chair all the way around, elevate the chair and wash dishes. It also helps a little at retrieving items from the shelves but not nearly so much as a GRABBER from Wal-Mart. If you ride with the seat up, it raises your center of gravity, thereby increasing risk of tipping. If you ride with the seat down your knees will protrude sideways and will kiss many door frames.

In the last 10 years, scooter manufacturers have blossomed. The quantity of scooters available far exceeds my research. I will give information on those with whom I have some familiarity and you can research many more by searching "mobility scooters" on Google.

The increased risk of tipping when riding a three wheel vs. a four wheel is rarely a consideration. Tipping over sideways can occur by leaning too far to the side, riding across a very steep slope, running over a large object on one side, or driving off a curb at an angle so that the wheel, or wheels on one side drop off much sooner than the other. These can cause tipping even on a four wheel if extreme enough. If you have difficulty deciding between three wheel or four wheel, maybe Rascal has your answer.

Goto:
http://www.rascalscooters.com/index.cfm/mobility/products.conver
tablelanding

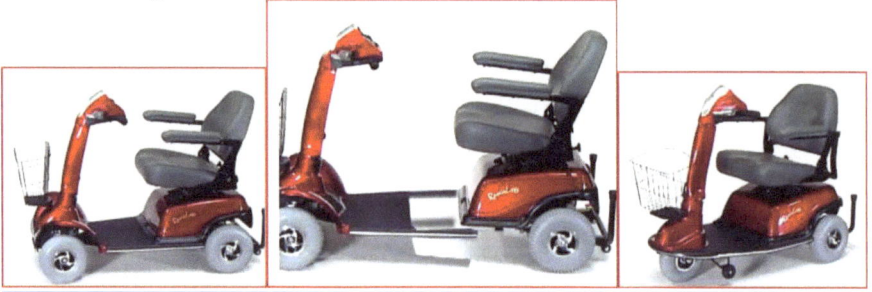

PRIDE SCOOTERS

I bought my Pride Victory 10 from, and can highly recommend:

http://www.healthunlimitedtexas.com

To shop and compare all Pride scooters, go to:

http://www.pridemobility.com/includes/download.php?f=brochures
/endtoend/ScooterEndtoEnd.pdf

The Amigo Scooter

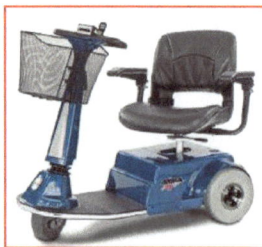

Similar to mine

Keeping Mobile on Your Scooter

http://www.gomobilityscooters.com/Amigo_Scooters_s/68.htm

http://www.Amazon.com, Offers Scooters reasonably priced and a nice selection.

http://www.scooter.com/
They have a big selection there.

http://www.scooterdirect.com/
This company seem to be priced reasonably.
They have many scooters, hoists, lift chairs, ramps etc. A lift chair helps me immensely when transferring out of my reclining lift chair and onto the scooter seat.

Keep ground clearance and ramp height in mind when purchasing or planning a scooter ramp.

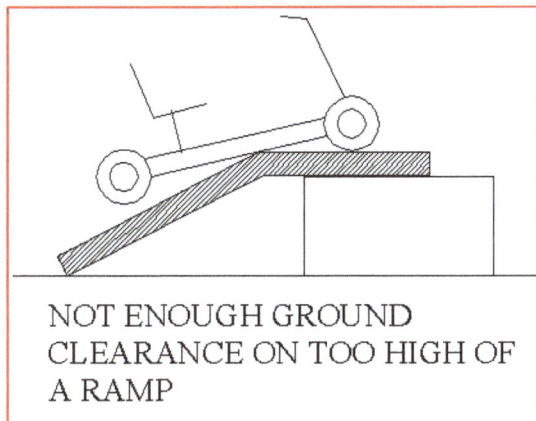

NOT ENOUGH GROUND CLEARANCE ON TOO HIGH OF A RAMP

Keeping Mobile on Your Scooter

I have a portable scooter ramp that weighs about 25 pounds. It is rated to carry 300 pounds on each of the two ramps. A scooter with four wheels can weigh up to 600 pounds total, including rider.

The maximum recommended angle for an unaided rider is 12:2, or a ramp going onto a 2 foot deck should be extend at least 12 feet along the ground. Steeper angles are acceptable with rider being assisted and if ground clearance is sufficient as seen in the above diagram.

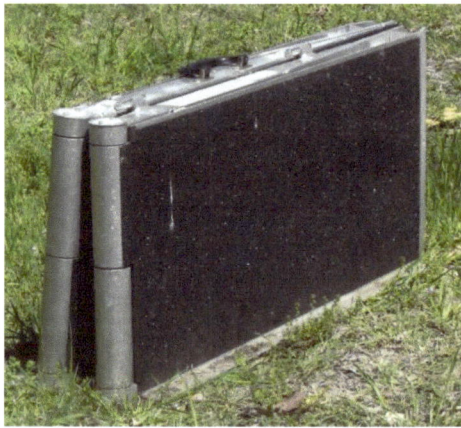

My portable ramps

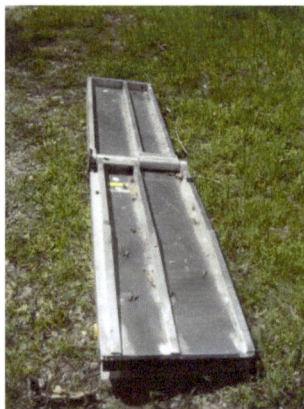

Ramps half open

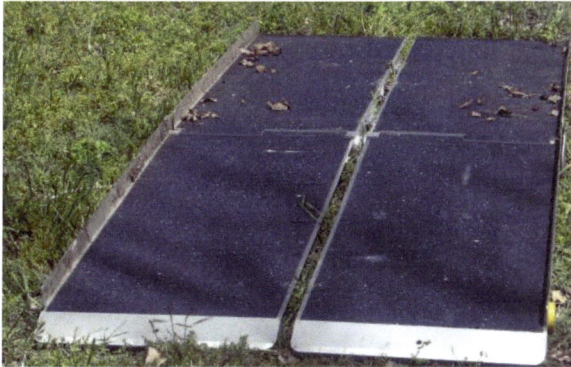

Ramps fully open (near end is top end)

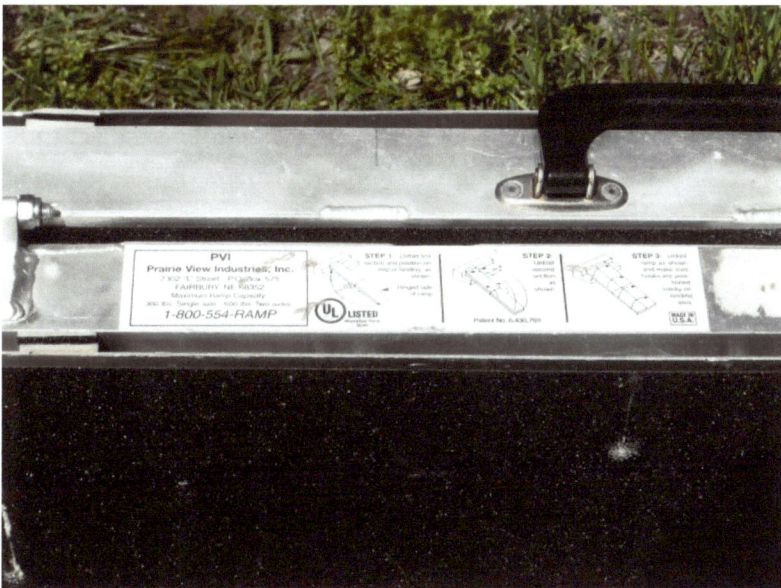

Ramps Label

CHAPTER 5
SCOOTERS I HAVE OWNED IN THE PAST

Chair type scooters can drive up to the dinner table with occupant seated normally. I have never felt it an imposition to drive alongside the table and rotate my seat to face the table.

Rascal 260 (ELECTRIC MOBILITY)

I bought my first scooter, a used Rascal about 1988 and also bought a really nice trailer for my wife to ride on when she had foot surgery. She did not have a severe mobility problem but was having difficulty keeping up with me on my wheels. That trailer was much more for fun than necessity.

The Rascal/Caboose trailer combination was too long going up and down in elevators. It had a tongue wheel so it could be wheeled like a wheelchair and take a different elevator than the scooter. I think the "Rascal Caboose" trailer went out of production 15 years ago but I just found one on EBAY for $150. I do not know its age.

Because of this inconvenience , my wife did not like it so she would sit in a wheelchair, catch my seat post with a cane and would "trailer" behind my scooter. Later she eliminated the cane and just held onto my scooter seat because she had much more directional control over her "trailering" wheelchair. We did and had no problems. I cannot recommend that you do this as I do not know your abilities.

Ann could walk but the Boardwalk in Atlantic City it was a challenge keeping up with my wheels.

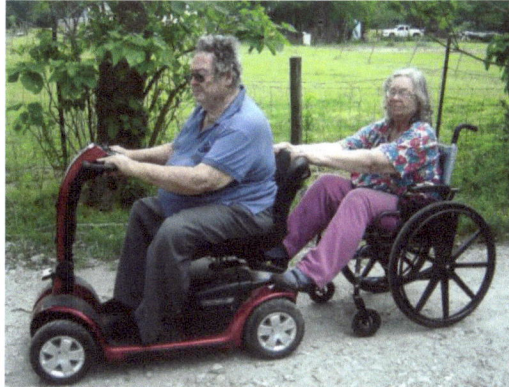

"Trailering" behind a scooter

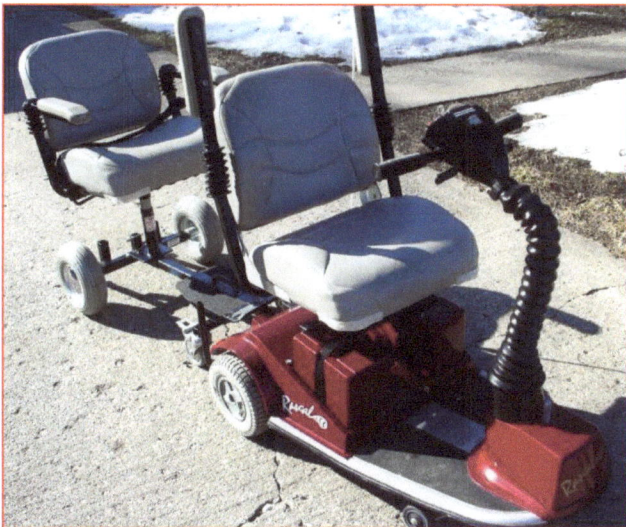

The Caboose trailer and my type of Rascal scooter.

When I could walk short distances I used my scooter indoors rarely and the Rascal was my favorite. It has an on board battery charger. This is the scooter with which I pulled the scooter trailer. Note the throttle paddle is in front of the handlebar and beyond accidental contact.

My Rascal ownership has been a pleasure, especially on rough roads. Be advised that it is slightly too large for most bathrooms.

I can say that in my many years of scooter ownership and riding, I have never found a "Bad" scooter. All give excellent service with battery replacement being the only near future expense.

PRIDE VICTORY 10

I purchased this scooter new in early 2010. It is a four wheeler with 40 AMP-HOUR batteries. It has a row of LED headlights that does fine and goes about 5 ¾ MPH. It is a power house. It is big and weighs about 200 lbs. I drive this one about ½ mile to church on Sundays. It is usually a pleasant drive. The Victory 10 is rather large when parked in the aisle but no one has tripped over it yet.

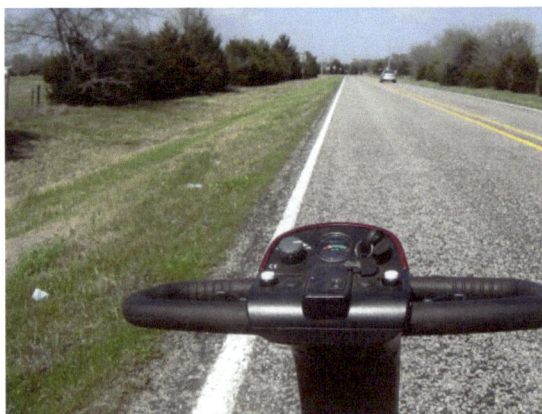

Going to Church on my Victory

In riding the Pride Victory 10 I can find very few faults with it. The big turning radius, of which I was aware before purchasing, makes it is too clumsy to even be very useful in the house. I measured 5.75 MPH with my GPS. It is an excellent outdoor scooter. It has independently sprung front wheels. Otherwise one wheel of a four wheel can go onto an obstruction, lifting that corner of the scooter and resulting in loss of ground traction.

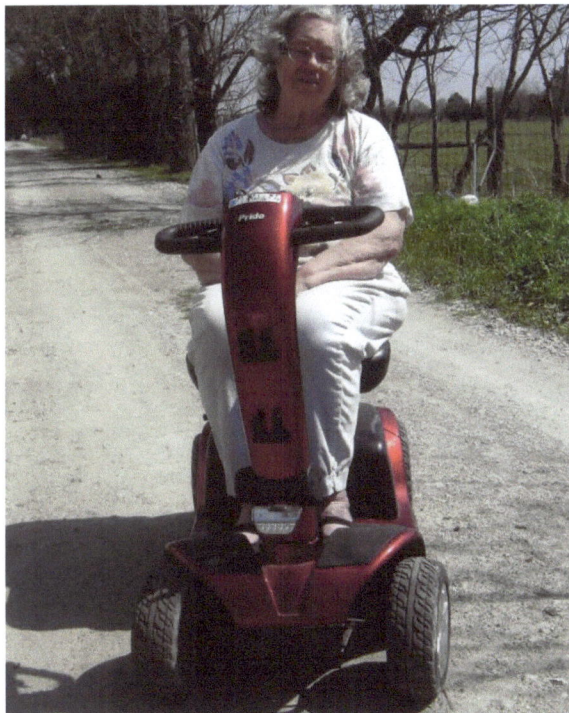

My wife, Ann on the Pride Victory 10,
When not gardening on it
(Basket and arm rests removed)

I also tried out the huge Pride Hurricane. It would just barely go through my front door and once inside it could not be moved about very easily. It would do 10 MPH. It was a blockage in the church aisle. That was a really fun scooter and very powerful but for outside only.

Pride Sonic

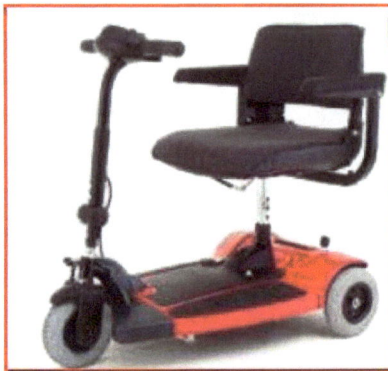

My Pride Sonic

I truly love my Pride Sonic 85 pound three wheel scooter. It is now awaiting a new battery wire. I took the batteries out to replace them, waited overnight and my cats made off with one of the 2 battery wires. I hear cats are "the other white meat" (kidding, I love our cats). The Sonic goes easily into my bathroom, *most* of the time.

> The Sonic is also a thumb-operated throttle with surprise movement when leaning forward and accidently striking the throttle paddle. I installed a push button key to make it easier to turn off and on. It saddens me that it is no longer in production. That is my main scooter when I go anywhere in my van or Buick. I load it, without disassembly, into the Nissan Quest Van using my Bruno Curbsider hoist, or with seat removed using my Bruno trunk hoist into the Buick trunk. It weighs 85 lbs. and has many miles on it. It has an on board battery charger.

MY CURBSIDER LOWERING MY RASCAL
SCOOTER TO CURB (SIDEWALK) POSITION.

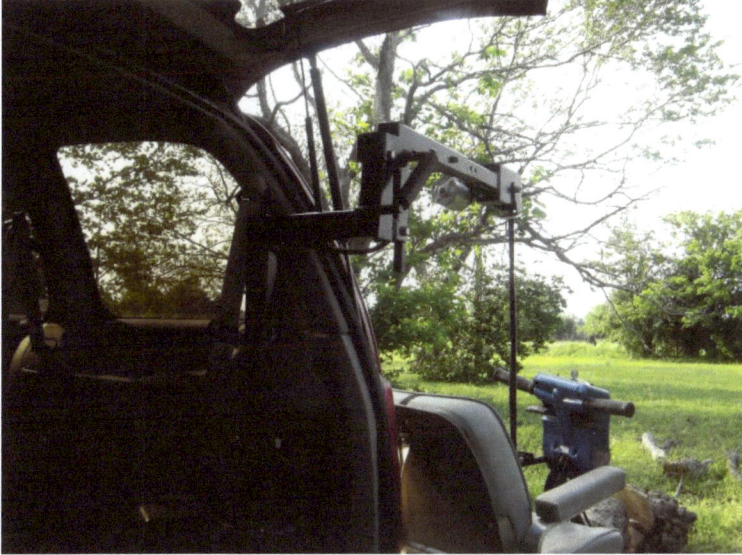

Hoist will fold down out of the way when not in use

What to check on a potential purchase

I do have only one negative to say about some of the scooters I have ridden. They LEAP! When slowly advancing the throttle, they will go maybe 3" immediately.

Conversely, you can put a dime in front of my Pride Sonic and I can stop it on dead center.

A personal note:

I just finished riding my Pride Victory about a mile, in the pleasant spring evening, to the cemetery. I drove effortlessly all around the grassy areas visiting gravesites of departed loved ones. A perfect scooter for that.
We had a small tornado hit us the other night and the Victory 10 headlights pierced the blackness at 3:00 AM. The scooter was easier to find in pitch blackness than a flashlight.

That scooter was very handy as damage surveying transportation: Front porch destroyed, 47 trees were damaged and 26 trees uprooted on 2 ½ acres.

The Amigo Scooter

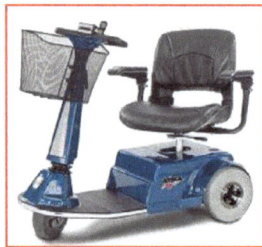

Similar to mine

I bought an Amigo scooter used. I loaned it to a friend who moved to New Orleans. My Amigo died in storage in Katrina floods.
It had a thumb operated throttle with the typical surprise starts when leaning forward and accidently moving the throttle. This is obviously correctable by turning off the ignition before leaning forward. Speed control at startup was good.
It had a retractable power cord built in. Very nice.

<u>Hoveround.com</u>- They have several types available. The chair type is controlled by joystick and can be driven right up a dining table in the eating position.

Even after all these years of riding, using the finger pull or thumb push throttles, I still occasionally command the wrong direction. The joystick makes it more intuitive.

Access Point Medical

My other Three wheel is an Access Point Medical. I bought it New on EBAY for $600, including shipping, in 2007. I then had two good insider Three wheelers. This scooter has a separate battery charger.

It is a good scooter but:

> I have some bad experience with **Access Point Medical**. The throttle return spring broke and they will not return my calls in my attempts to get a new one. My scooter is now using a rubber band on forward throttle and a balancing rubber band on backward throttle. Without these rubber bands, it is a suicide machine, full forward or full backward as it desires. See picture.

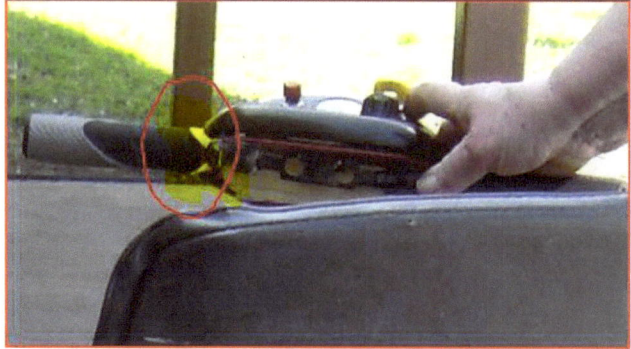

RUBBER BAND ON THROTTLE LEVER
OF MY
ACCESS POINT MEDICAL SCOOTER

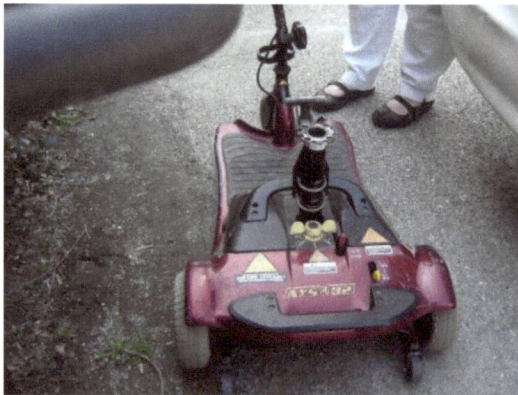

My Access Point Medical before installing seat.

DALTON (16 ½" wide)

This is a scooter on loan from John, noted in my dedication. It goes
through the bathroom door with ease. It has 2 narrowly spaced

front wheels and is longer than either of my small Three wheelers. Turning in the hallway outside of the bathroom is a tricky maneuver since it is longer than my other three wheelers. It has a separate battery charger. I use it in the house so my wife will not have to unload the three wheeler Sonic from the car every time we return home.

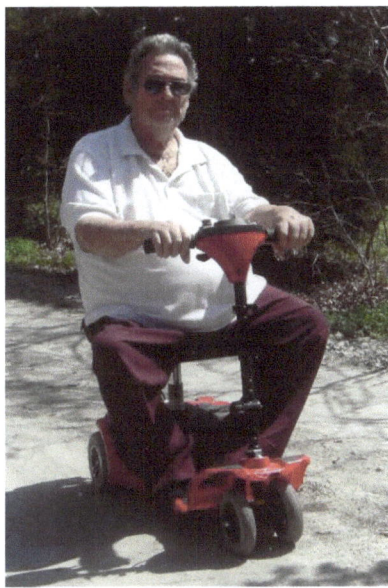

The Dalton

Hoveround

(A drive up to the table type scooter)

I bought a used Hoveround because of its advertised maneuverability. It was a nice solid and comfortable scooter with a joystick control. The main wheels were directly below the rider and it had trailer wheels in the rear. To turn LEFT, the trailer wheels would go to the RIGHT as the chair rotated. It was a challenge to remember to allow room for turning without impacting the wall. There are a lot of scooters out there with this design so it is not rare. It is the picture on the left. The picture on the right is their three wheel design that does not swing when turning.

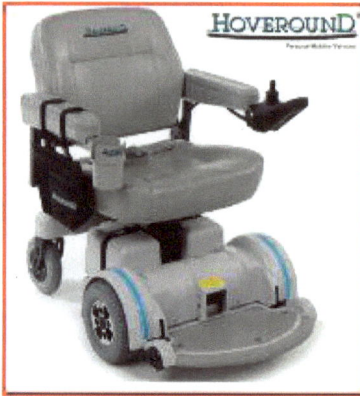

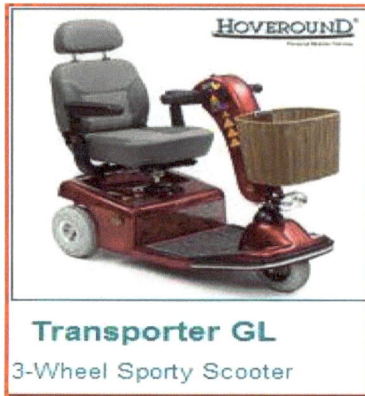

This is my objection to scooters with trailer wheels in back

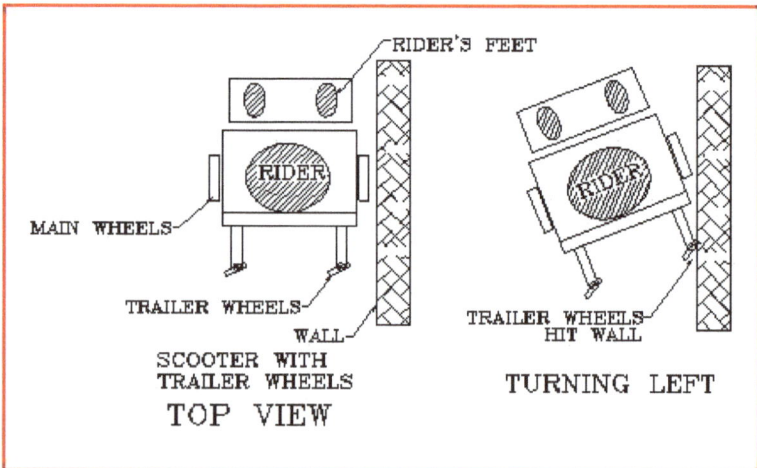

TRAILER WHEELS STRIKING WALL WHEN TURNING.

CHAPTER 6
TRAVELING WTH AND/OR TRANSPORTING A HANDICAP SCOOTER

Be advised that Medicare will pay only for a scooter required by you INDOORS. When it comes time to travel outside the home, assistive equipment, such as hoists, transfer boards, ramps etc. is out of your pocket. As noted elsewhere, when I applied for Medicare assistance on a $1,000 lifting chair recliner, they said "you buy it and maybe we will reimburse up to 35%". Many automobile lifts and hoists are available at the big name scooter manufacturers and distributors.

The name "lift" and "hoist" are many times used interchangeably. A hoist is generally an item that has strap with a hook , or other means of scooter attachment at the end and when attached to the scooter, it "hoists" it into the air. A lift usually supports the scooter on its wheels and then raises it.

Your choices in taking a scooter with you when travelling are:

By your personal vehicle:

1. Disassemble scooter into front, rear, seat and batteries. Load individual parts into vehicle. Most normal size scooters will fit into most normal size cars. Always remember to take the battery charger with you. Parts latch together at arrival but with some alignment difficulty.

2. By removing the scooter seat and folding the handlebar down, it can be loaded into a trunk using a trunk hoist.

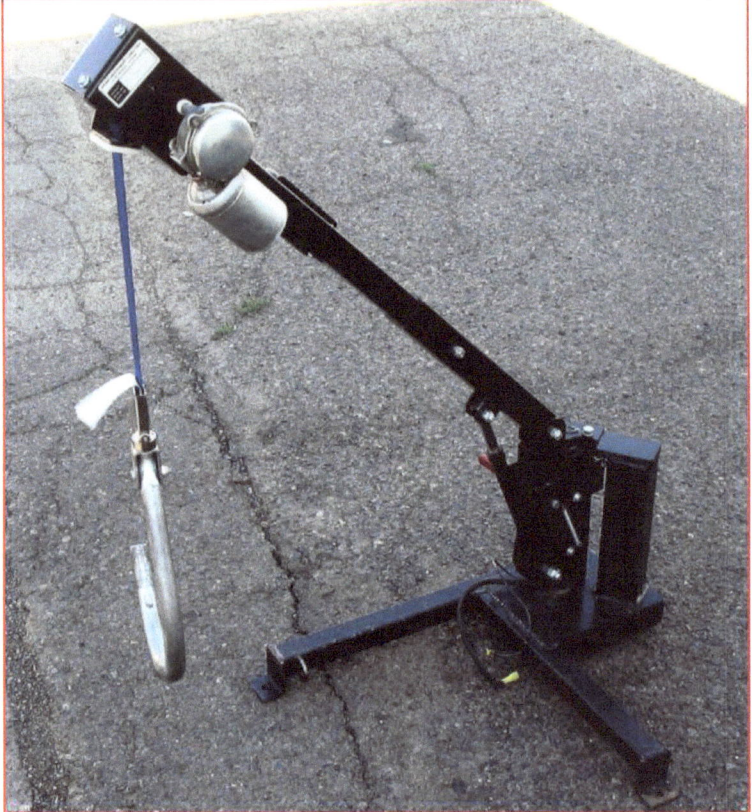

A Bruno trunk hoist (Later model than mine, and does not require disassembly of hoist after use.)

Note that my Rascal 260 is too big for my Buick trunk using the lift. It must be disassembled and loaded piece by piece. Most normal three wheelers will fit fine by the hoist. The scooter must have a "T BAR" mounted to the seat post. All hoists have a slotted claw that fits onto the T bar and winds up with the attaching hoisting belt.

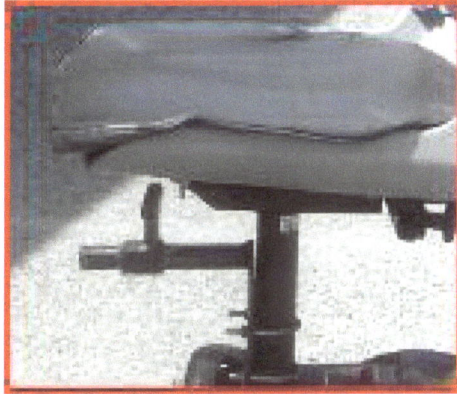

T Bar

3. If you have a Van, you can install a swing out hoist. I installed a Bruno Curbsider into a Suburban and later transferred it to a '96 Nissan Quest. It would load and unload a completely assembled scooter from the rear or from the adjacent curb.

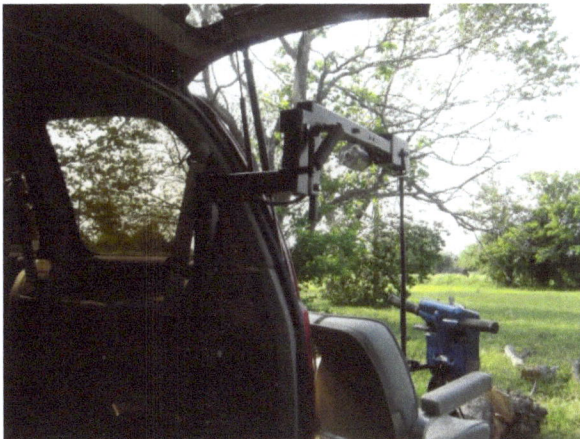

4. If you have a strong trailer hitch, you can have a scooter platform on the ground to drive the scooter onto. The hoist frame is inserted in the trailer hitch receptacle like a trailer

hitch. The scooter is lifted and secured at the back bumper while travelling. Note that this offers no weather protection for the scooter. Remember that rain blows up from below when driving. It also adds to the length of the vehicle when the scooter is loaded.

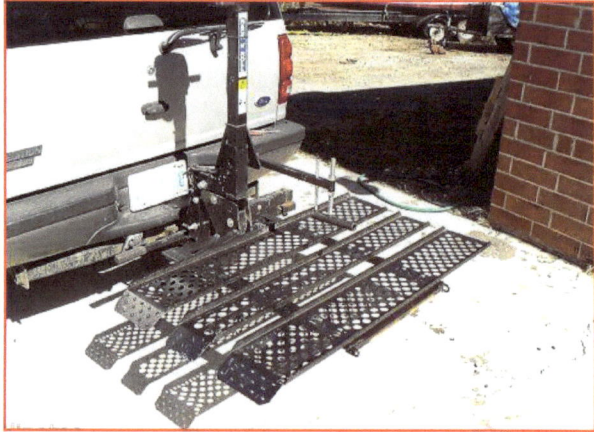

Many designs will fold the lift upward when a scooter is not loaded, to minimize length of vehicle.

5. You can purchase water proof covers custom made from the scooter manufacturer.
    A friend had a scooter friendly shower built in his home and would ride his covered three wheel Amigo into the shower for bathing.

6. My situation is such that I cannot walk from the back of the vehicle to the driver's door so after getting off of the scooter and into the car, my wife takes the scooter around to the back and loads it into the trunk, or into the Van.

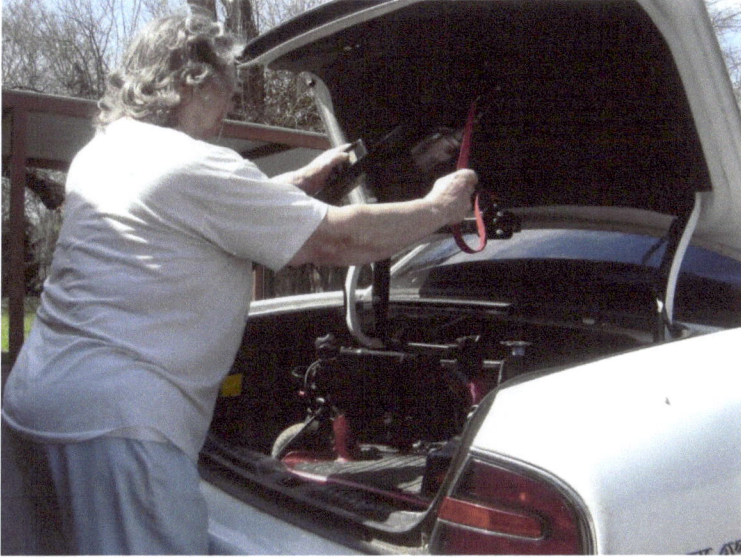

7. Of course, the ultimate would be a van with a wheelchair lift. May times these are designed to allow the wheelchair occupant to get into position to drive while still in the wheelchair.

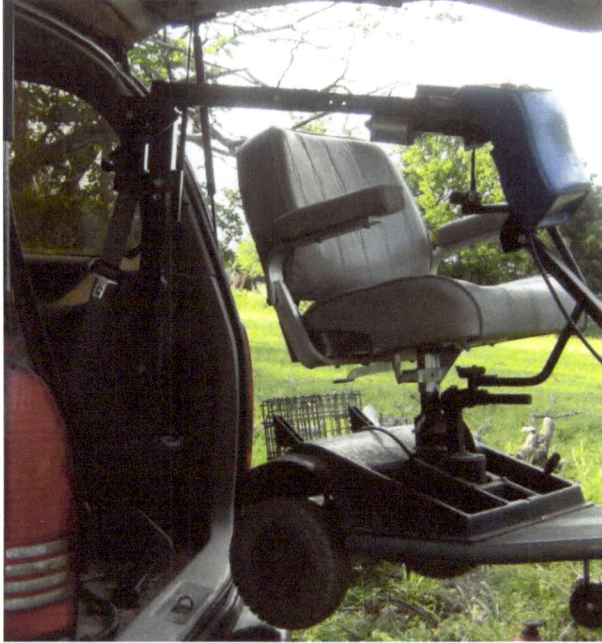

BRUNO CURBSIDER HOIST
SHOWING T BAR AND CLAW
LIFTING MY RASCAL SCOOTER

As noted previously:

<u>Airline Travel</u>: I have travelled by air many times with my 138 pound Rascal, three wheel or my 85 pound Sonic three wheel. Usually you can ride down the jet way to the aircraft door. From there, you either walk to your seat or they take you in a narrow aisle wheelchair.

Then they take your scooter down the jet way stairway to be put into the baggage area. They are not responsible for damage although I have never had any serious damage.

When I get to my destination, sometime they take the scooter to baggage claim, whereupon they will wheelchair you to baggage claim. Other times, they will meet you at the door of the plane. There is no extra charge to take the scooter. DON'T FORGET YOUR CHARGER.

CHAPTER 7

RIDING AND SAFETY TIPS

Do not fear the three wheel scooter tipping over sideways. It is an extremely rare occurrence.

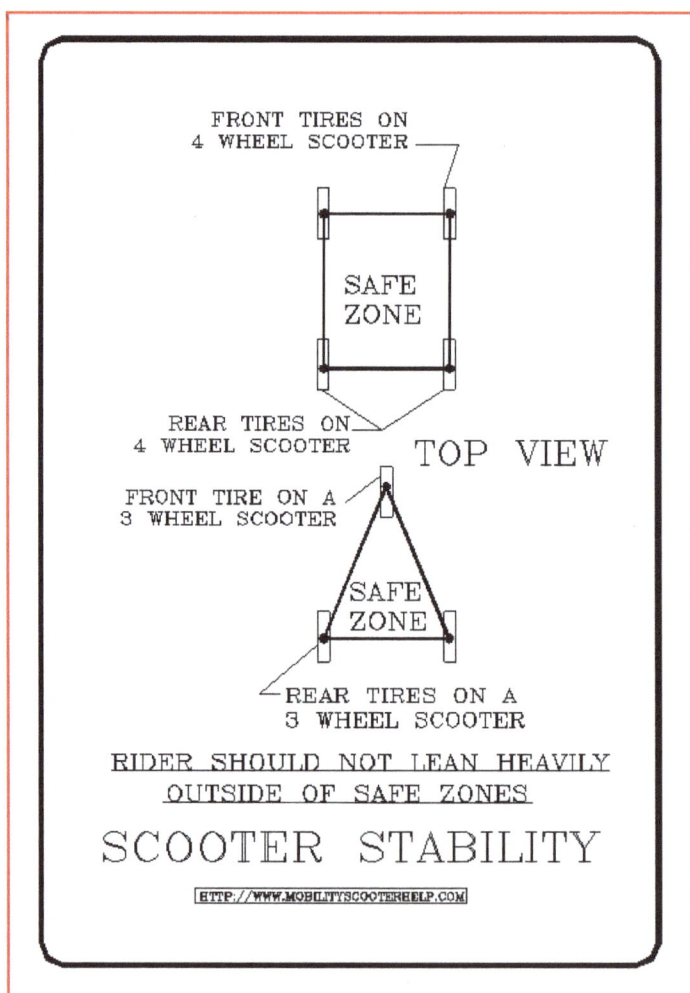

Keeping Mobile on Your Scooter

<u>Now what to look for in a scooter</u>:

1. A small scooter with a width of less than 22 inches. A three wheel will be much more maneuverable. This scooter will also serve outside in firm terrain. The weight would be less than 100 lbs which is appreciated by airline personnel when flying.
2. Most scooters disassemble into four parts.
   a. Rear drive assembly-30 to 48 lbs
   b. Front forks assembly about 25-40 lbs
   c. Seat-about 20 lbs and
   d. Batteries- about 20 lbs.
3. These parts can be placed in the trunk of most cars for travel. Disassembly is easy but reassembly is a little trickier, more a game of positioning parts.
4. If you select a three wheel scooter, it is diagrammed above that it can be tipped over sideways by leaning too far. A four wheel scooter is more resistant to tipping. Since 1988, one time I forgot that I had transferred from my four wheel to my three wheel. I leaned too far and tipped sideways.
5. Road speeds can be from 3 1/2 MPH to about 5 ½ MPH for normal scooters. There are some that will travel 10 MPH or more but that is usually not necessary, and it increases the danger of tipping over sideways in a sudden turn.
6. Four wheel scooters generally do better in travelling in the yard. I learned the hard way that pea gravel will bog you down instantly on any scooter.
7. A smaller scooter should have 2 each 12 Amp-Hour batteries.
8. My bigger scooters have 32 Amp-hour and my big four wheel Pride has 40 Amp-hour batteries.

Most scooters with 12 AMP-HOUR batteries will go about 7-15 miles between charges and my Pride scooter, with 40 AMP-HOUR batteries will go up to 28 miles.

My Rascal scooter weighs about 135 lbs with 2 ea 32 AMP-HOUR (U1) batteries. I climbed Mount Rainer to the end of the foot path on it. It explored Hawaii a day longer than I did, thanks to airline baggage errors.

In the TV commercial, when you see the ladies on the rim of Grand Canyon on their Hoverounds, You can bet your bottom dollar that the scooters were placed there and the batteries disconnected, because....

Even after all these years, I still use the wrong throttle paddle, going forward when I meant to go backward.
So many times, I have stopped to get something and in reaching for it, I accidentally leaned across the backward throttle causing my scooter to leap backward in a dangerous manner. My Rascal has the throttles on the front side of the handle bars to be pulled by a finger. It has never moved accidently. My Pride Victory has the throttles protected and can be pushed with the thumb or pulled with the finger.

The instruction manuals caution you to turn off the ignition when stopped. What a bore! The most ridiculous thing to be found on scooters is a button for a "Horn". The horn is a pitiful chirp and the mouth of the rider is plenty close to people in the way to simply say: "Excuse me" The backing up horn will drive you up the wall.

I have replaced this horn button with a push-on, push-off button for instantaneous on-off on all my scooters. The key switch can be left in the circuit to lock against unauthorized use.

Keeping Mobile on Your Scooter

In case you are handy with a soldering iron, or have a friend who is, here is how to convert your scooter to using a push button for on/off. It will probably cancel your warrantee so wait until it expires.

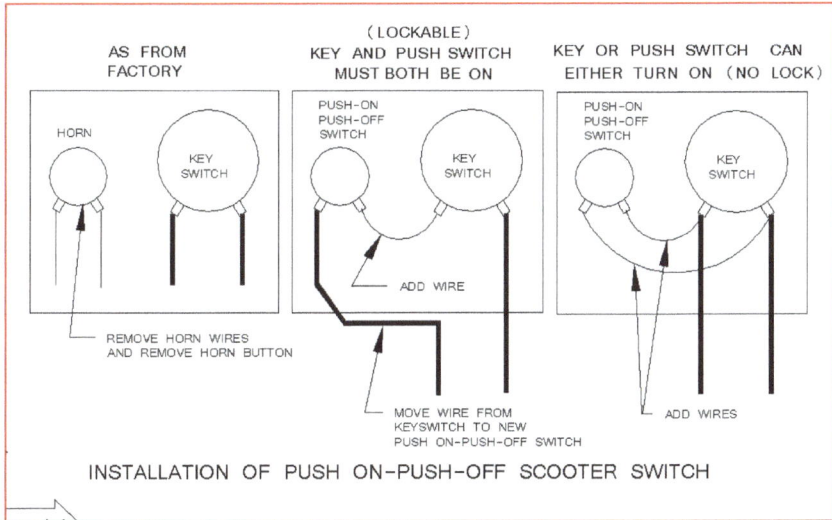

INSTALLATION OF PUSH ON-PUSH-OFF SCOOTER SWITCH

You can probably get a push-on, push-off switch at Radio Shack. Amperage is low.

Safety tips

Roadway Operation:

Always ride on the left, facing traffic. Be aware that most drivers will give you a wide berth **UNLESS** there is traffic meeting him.

WHEN SOMEONE IS COMING TOWARD YOU FROM THE FRONT AND YOU HEAR TRAFFIC

COMING FROM BEHIND TOWARD HIM, STOP OFF THE ROADWAY AND LET THEM PASS. THE ONE COMING TOWARD YOU CANNOT GIVE YOU EXTRA SAFETY ROOM.

Use a tall flag and/or reflective tape on your scooter.

Advice:

Don't challenge motorcycles to a race "title for title". What would you do with a motorcycle if you won it?

When riding across a slope, you can lean uphill for more stability.

When going up a hill drive a serpentine path to ease the load on the drive motor.

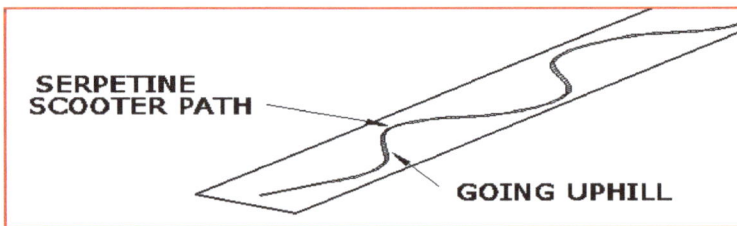

SERPETINE SCOOTER PATH

GOING UPHILL

A REAL CAUTION

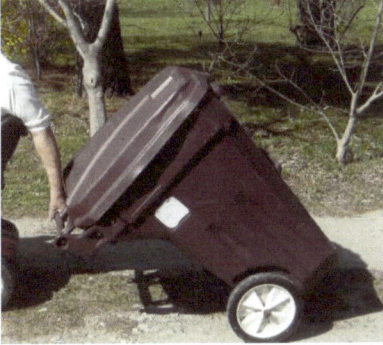

When pulling a load with a hand, keep your hand low.

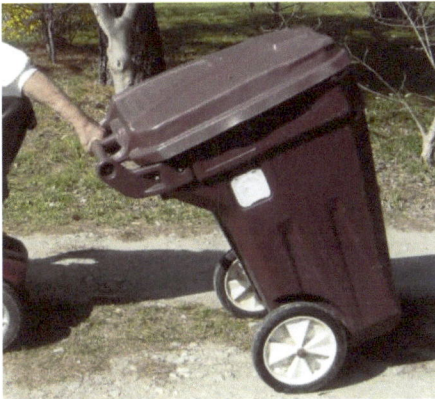

Pulling with your hand high can tip you over backward.

CHAPTER 8

SCOOTER CARE

Your scooter will give years of service without much attention. Not so for batteries. Battery replacement can be from $50 to $250. It makes good sense to take good care of them. A well cared for battery can last 2 years or longer. If qualified by Medicare, battery replacement and service is covered.

Never leave your batteries in the run down condition. Use only the charger that came with the scooter, usually about a 2 amp charge. After batteries are fully charged, remove charger. Do not leave batteries charging any longer than necessary to return to full charge.

It is always wise to replace batteries in pairs. They are connected in "series" meaning the negative of one battery is connected to the positive of the other battery, thereby totaling the voltage i.e. 12 Volts plus 12 Volts equals 24 volts, as used by the scooter.

A problem with the normal arrangement is that during charging, the stronger of the two batteries will not charge well because of the weaker battery being in the circuit.

Even if not being used, recharge batteries at least once a month, but not continuously.

CHAPTER 9

FINANCING HANDICAP SCOOTERS (As of 2011)

My only knowledge here is what I have experienced and that is;

A big scooter distributor can give much good help!

- Medicare will pay 80% of your scooter for indoor use. A Medigap policy usually pays the rest.
- I have been told by Medicare: "You buy it and we *MIGHT* reimburse 80%." when I tried to buy a new lift chair. I kept my old one.
- Medicare will not pay for a scooter used to go to the Doctor or other outside uses.
- Medicare will not pay for scooter hoisting equipment for your car.
- **If you have a licensed person install scooter and wheelchair equipment into your vehicle, Texas will forgive sales taxes on the vehicle purchase.**
- You can contact large distributors of scooters and they will try very hard to get you approved.
- When Medicare buys you a scooter, they will provide battery replacement at no charge.
- You must get a prescription from a Doctor saying that you are "Orthopedically handicapped" and not a suitable candidate for a wheelchair due to lack of arm mobility or strength."

CHAPTER 10

DISCUSSION AND TIPS

- You can widen any doorway 2 inches by replacing the existing hinges with "Offset" hinges that swing the door flush with the door jam.

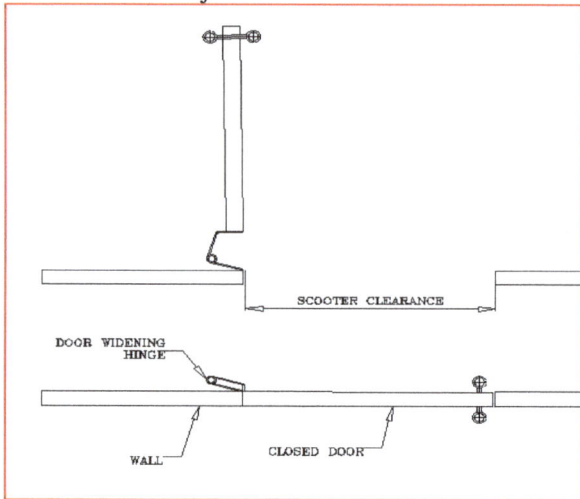

SCOOTER CLEARANCE

DOOR WIDENING HINGE

WALL   CLOSED DOOR

- These attractive and durable wheelchair door hinges allow you to open the door up completely flush with the wall, or allow you to open a door so it's completely flat and tucked away; up to a 180 degree swing. This helps remove that portion of the door that normally gets in the way of the passageway. The Expandable Offset Door Hinges adds 2" to any doorway opening to allow barrier free access for most wheelchairs or walkers. They are ideal for most bathroom doors and can be easily installed as they use the same screws and holes as the existing hinge. 3 holes, 2" x 3-1/2"

  http://www.sportaid.com/expandable-offset-door-hinges.html

Scooter problems:

Your point of purchase business will usually have a well-qualified technician to perform all service on your scooter.

Other than dead battery, the most problems I have had are with the switch attached to the brake lever.
If you try to drive the scooter and it will not go, but showing good battery charge, chances are the lever is in the **ROLL** position. In that position, the motor will not drive.

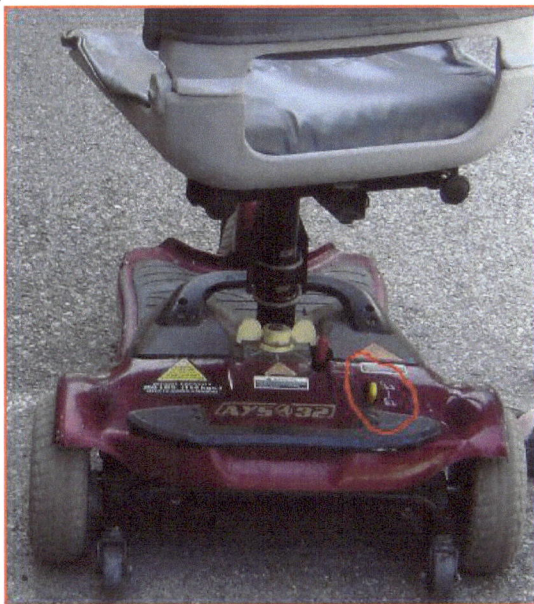

Brake lever must be in the drive position to ride.
In the rolling position it is free-wheeling with no brakes or motor.

The scooter also will not drive while the charging plug is connected to the scooter.

If neither situation is the problem, the chances are good that the micro-switch on the roll/drive lever is bad. Not an expensive part is somewhat difficult to access.

Getting on and off the Scooter.

I have a lift chair that lifts me to seat height and I just slide across. (Search "lift chair" on the internet.)
If you have difficulty transferring to a chair or car, I highly suggest a transfer board. I used a borrowed one during an unusual physical requirement. There are various prices but the one I borrowed had a travelling roller seat and is more expensive.

Be sure to check out a "boogie board" for use to transfer from bed to wheelchair, wheelchair to bath and wheelchair to automobile. The Beasy Transfer Boards use a frictionless bearing system for smooth, easy sliding with swivel a seat for greatest flexibility.
http://www.phc-online.com/Transfer_Boards_s/124.htm

Rain protection

Electric scooters do not like water. Avoid driving through puddles or in the rain.

Scooter theft

Don't get too complacent about leaving your scooter unattended. A healthy man can easily pick up a locked scooter and put it in a vehicle.

Arm Rests

Most scooter arm rests are easily removable. That is the first thing I remove. My Rascal arm rests are not easily removable but swing up out of the way .

Baskets

The front basket support on the Rascal is mounted to the frame and not the front forks. The basket load remains still when turning the forks. You will notice my photo of an optional rear basket. It mounts to the seat frame and is very sturdy. All baskets are removable. **When grocery shopping, I simply pull a shopping cart behind me. They follow well. I can leave it while gathering other nearby things.**

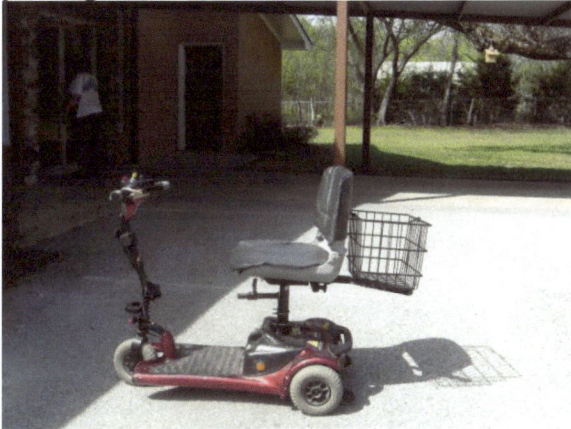

My rear basket inserts into the seat frame receptacle

Throttle bar

You will notice on the picture of Rascal, the throttle paddle is in front of the handle grips. No chance of accidental acceleration when leaning over.

Joystick

The joystick controls forward, backward left and right. The brakes are on when it is in center position and not driving.

Battery replacement

Many of today's scooters now have both batteries in a single removable case. This makes it easier to remove when separating the scooter into separate parts for car travel

The following pictures show the replacement of batteries inside of a containing case:

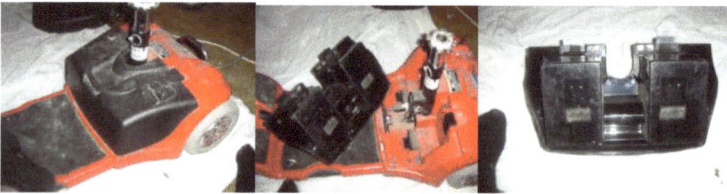

Remove screws from bottom and set upright

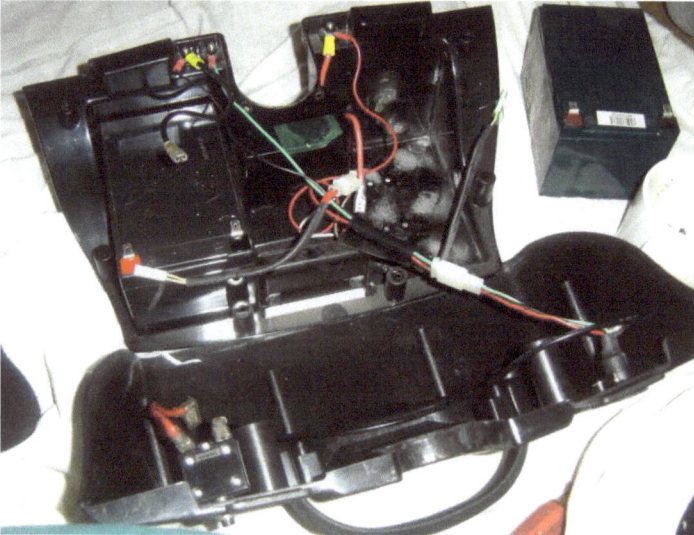

- Lift off top, unplug slide on clips from battery terminals

- Lift out old batteries. Insert new batteries
- Push on slide on clips observing red and black markings
- Put top back on.
- Turn upside down and replace screws.

How most scooter drive systems operate

- With the key off, battery is off and automatic brakes are on.

- When key is turned on, power is applied to the scooter control system and the throttle or joystick is being monitored for movement requests.

- Pressing a throttle paddle or tilting the joystick causes the brakes to release and drive to occur in the desired direction.

- Speed of travel is controlled by the amount of throttle, or joystick, movement.

- Direction of movement is by the handlebars or the left/right component of the leaning of the joystick

- All throttle controls will return back to the neutral position by just releasing,. That will cause the motor to stop driving and the brakes to apply.

- It is recommended that the power switch be turned off while getting on, or off. Accidental contact with the throttle when you are only half on can be quite hazardous.

- If you are pressing a throttle paddle when turning on the key, it will not turn on the electronics. The key must be turned completely off, release the throttle and then turn the key on. A good safety feature but it has cost me time when in a real hurry by getting the throttle ahead of the switch.

- Another quirk of the drive systems is that it will shut down anytime the energy demand from the batteries causes a low battery voltage. With healthy batteries and at least a medium charge, this seldom happens. When you extend use with a low battery, it takes less and less rolling resistance to shut it down. Then you have to **turn it off, then on.**

- Inactivity will result in the scooter going into the sleep mode. You must **turn it off and then on** to move.

- Each scooter has a speed control. That control reduces sensitivity of the throttle position, i.e. instead of 4MPH max, with the speed control turned down; full throttle may be only ½ MPH. Turning this control down also limits demands on your battery and could extend travel before the next automatic shutdown from low battery.

- The rear axle usually has a differential drive like your car. The brakes lock the automobile equivalent of the drive shaft and NOT individual wheels. The scooter can be tilted to lift one rear wheel from the floor when being moved by a walking person. The wheel in the air is free to turn the other direction from the one on the floor. Like your car, the scooter will not drive out of a soft area if one wheel is free to spin.

- **This gives rise to a caution about scooter brakes:** On slippery ground, or with one wheel on slippery ground such as ice or mud, you have minimum brakes. **If one wheel has poor traction, the other wheel will not provide any braking effect, even though on solid ground.** Your car has brakes on each wheel, not so scooters.

KEEP YOUR BATTERIES CHARGED BUT NOT CONSTANTELY.

Battery chargers emit some radio interference. They are usually not too bad in this field.

Solar Battery Charging

An interesting concept is to have solar panels charging your scooter batteries. This would be a clumsy approach to make portable, but if unusual circumstances occurred; no home electricity or gas for your car is available, it may be your only choice to keep your scooter mobile and charged. A home solar array panel of 24 volts, 2 to 5 amps would make you independent (50 to120 watts) of civilization and would be quite pratical. This would require tapping into the scooter battery terminals. Otherwise, a solar array of about 200 watts with a converter to convert the solar panel DC to 115 volts AC would be a simple-plug in for your scooter charger. This power source could prove valuable elsewhere too.

My only financial connection in this book is my Solar Panels website where you will find a solar panel build-it-yourself book:

www.easy-diy-solar.com

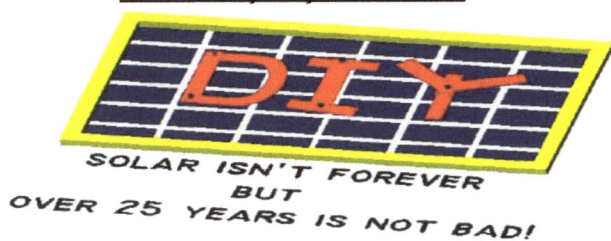

SOLAR ISN'T FOREVER BUT OVER 25 YEARS IS NOT BAD!

If you have the money and can afford to purchase industrial solar panels, you will find DIY a lot of trouble, but consider what a thrilling task that would be for the scooter occupant. A lot of sitting and soldering. A little assistance by a person able to walk could be beneficial when handling completed panels.

A 12 VDC to 115 VAC converter in your car can operate your charger, but will quickly run the batteries down in a non-running car. This can be a good answer while driving.

It is possible to attach an accessory receptacle (Cigarette lighter) to one battery to provide charging for your cell phone, laptop, etc. Avoid excessive use from one battery by attaching a second receptacle to the other and exchanging usage occasionally.
These can also provide access to one battery at a time for charging each battery using a 12 volt charger. Minor charging current could be from a 12 VDC solar panel automobile battery maintenance panel. DO NOT WIRE ACROSS BOTH BATTERIES. This would result in 24 volts and destroy anything plugged into the accessory receptacle.

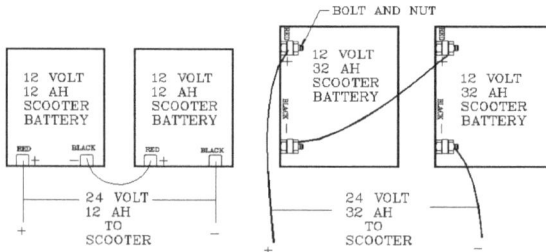

BATTERY CONNECTIONS IN SCOOTERS

Keeping Mobile on Your Scooter

ABOUT THE AUTHOR

MY BIO

My name is Morris Barwick and I am a retired mechanical engineer. My degree is from the **University of Florida.**

I had Poliomyelitis in the late '30's (before vaccines) and have had to wear a full leg brace all my life. However, I rarely let it limit my activities. I owned a 5-mile paper route as a kid, which I threw from a bicycle. I have been a private pilot for many years, with more than 300 hours as "Pilot in Command". I owned my own airplane, a Piper Cherokee 140 (hand operated brakes are standard).

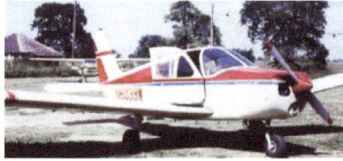

My professional career was largely composed of consulting engineering which included the design of rockets, spacesuits, and electronics in the "Space Race" and military.

I didn't know that my years of relatively carefree activity was slowly coming to an end, and with the late onset of Post-Polio Syndrome, I would soon be scooter bound.

In previous years, the only option for me would be a wheelchair , or an electric wheelchair. These were very expensive, confining, cumbersome, and not very versatile. When the new electric mobility scooters started to appear, the appeal was overwhelming.

Keeping Mobile on Your Scooter

A person with limited mobility had many more options that were more appealing than before. I have known many elderly people who were embarrassed and ashamed to admit they needed a wheelchair (and usually someone else to push it), Many times they would deny themselves outings where limited mobility might be a problem.

Since I bought my first scooter in 1988, I have had a professional fascination with them and in later years that fascination became a dependency. I have made an intensive study of mobility scooters and riding requirements. At one time Electric Mobility, manufacturer of the Rascal Scooter, requested my resume in anticipation of my providing design services to their firm. Regrettably the circumstances were not possible at that time.

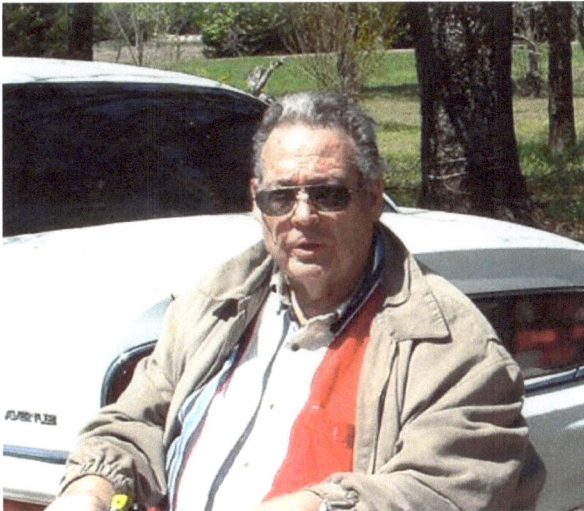

Morris Barwick
Feedback and Keeping in touch is appreciated at:
www.mobilityscooterclub.com